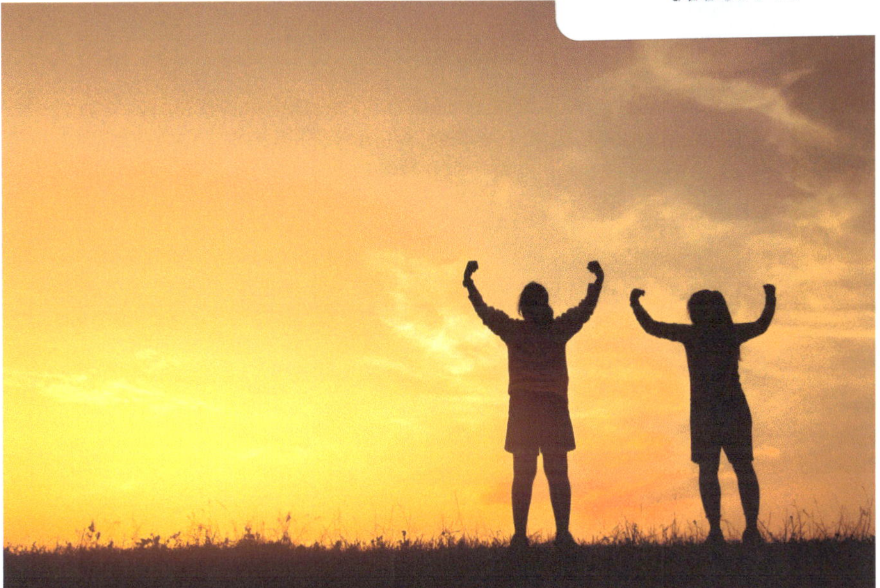

You're Already on Your Way!

At least once in our lifetime we've all woken up one morning and said to ourselves, "today is the day I will start my journey to becoming fit!" This initiative usually begins well as we're determined to succeed and reach our goals. Plus, we receive great advice from friends & family and social media posts which further boosts our confidence. However, after a some time, we begin to question our efforts and lack of results when looking in the mirror. We begin losing stamina and our desire to continue begins to wane. Sound familiar?? Well if this is true, our 1-2-3 guidebook is here to keep you motivated and excited about the journey to a fitter you. If you're disciplined and follow our coordinated step-by-step process, you may eventually be the one giving the fitness advice and posting your successes on social media! This book is meant to guide you through this process and to propel you to achieving your goals. At the end of of the book, you'll have a weekly planner to help keep you on track with your goals, exercise program, and nutritional plan. Be specific with your plan so you train your mind to be disciplined and results-driven. Wishing you the best of luck and remember if you do not believe in yourself, no one will do it for you.

BELIEVE IN YOU!

Action Plan

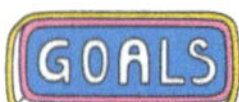

1.Set Clear Goals: Define specific, realistic, and achievable goals for your health and fitness journey. Whether it's weight loss, muscle gain, or improved endurance, having clear objectives will keep you focused.

2. Create a Plan: Develop a structured plan that includes both exercise and nutrition. Consider consulting with a fitness professional to tailor a program that suits your fitness level, preferences, and lifestyle.

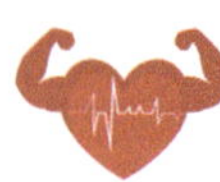

3. Mix Cardio and Strength Training: Include a combination of cardiovascular exercises (e.g., walking, running, cycling) and strength training (body weight is great to start) to enhance overall fitness. This variety keeps your workouts interesting and targets different aspects of health.

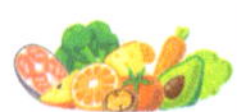

4. Prioritize Nutrition: Pay attention to your diet by incorporating whole foods, lean proteins, fruits, vegetables, and whole grains. Stay hydrated and consider consulting a nutritionist for personalized advice.

5. Schedule Regular Workouts: Consistency is key. Schedule regular workout sessions and treat them like appointments. Find a time that fits your daily routine and make it a habit.

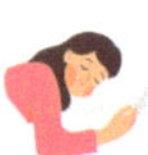

6. Get Enough Rest: Allow your body to recover by ensuring adequate sleep. Recovery is crucial for muscle repair and overall well-being.

7. Track Your Progress: Keep a record of your workouts, dietary habits, and any changes in your body. Tracking progress helps you stay motivated and makes it easier to identify areas for improvement.

8. Stay Positive and Patient: Understand that results take time. Celebrate small victories, stay positive, and be patient with the process. Consistency is more important than rapid progress.

Consider Professional Guidance: If possible, seek guidance from fitness professionals, such as personal trainers or health coaches. They can provide personalized advice, correct your form, devise an appropriate nutritional plan, and motivate you along the way.

Chapter 1: Setting Clear Goals for Your Health and Fitness Journey

Embarking on a health and fitness program is an exciting and transformative journey. However, before you dive into workouts and nutritional plans, it's essential to set clear and well-defined goals. Goals act as a roadmap, guiding your efforts and providing direction for your fitness endeavors. In this chapter, we'll explore the importance of setting goals and how to establish them effectively.

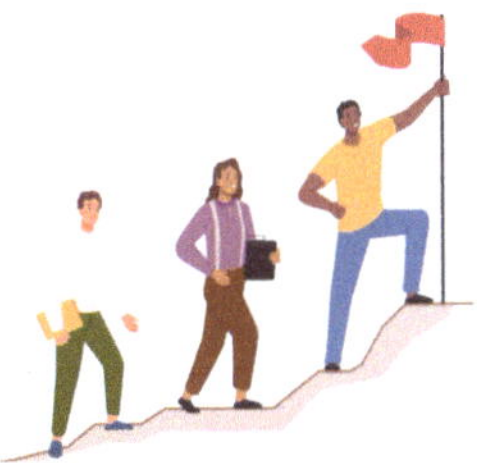

The Significance of Clear Goals

1. **Motivation and Focus**: Clear goals serve as powerful motivators. When you have a specific objective in mind, it becomes easier to stay focused on your fitness journey. Whether it's losing a certain amount of weight, building muscle, or improving endurance, having a target gives your efforts purpose.

2. **Measurable Progress:** Goals should be measurable, allowing you to track your progress over time. Tangible benchmarks help you celebrate achievements and adjust your approach if necessary. Regular assessments provide a sense of accomplishment and keep you on track.

3. **Personalization**: Your fitness goals should be tailored to your individual needs and desires. A personalized approach ensures that your program aligns with your preferences, making it more enjoyable and sustainable in the long run.

4. **Overcoming Plateaus**: In any fitness journey, there may be times when progress seems slow or even stagnant. Well-defined goals act as beacons during such periods, guiding you through plateaus and preventing discouragement.

How to Establish Clear Goals

1. **Be Specific**: Vague goals like "get fit" or "eat healthier" lack the specificity needed for effective planning. Instead, define your objectives clearly. For instance, aim to lose 10 pounds, run a 5K, or reduce body fat percentage by a certain amount.

2. **Set Realistic Targets**: While ambition is admirable, setting unrealistic goals can lead to frustration. Consider your current fitness level, lifestyle, and commitments. Establish targets that challenge you but remain achievable within a reasonable timeframe.

3. **Short-Term and Long-Term Goals**: Break down your overarching fitness goal into smaller, manageable targets. Short-term goals provide stepping stones, keeping you motivated with frequent achievements. Long-term goals offer a broader perspective, maintaining a sense of purpose throughout the journey.

4. **Include Behavioral Goals**: It's not just about the outcome; focus on behavioral goals as well. For example, commit to exercising four times a week, preparing a healthy meal each day, or getting sufficient sleep. These habits contribute to the overall success of your fitness journey.

5. **Write Them Down**: Document your goals using the weekly planning guide at the end of this book. Putting your goals in writing makes them tangible and reinforces your commitment. Regularly revisit and revise them as needed.

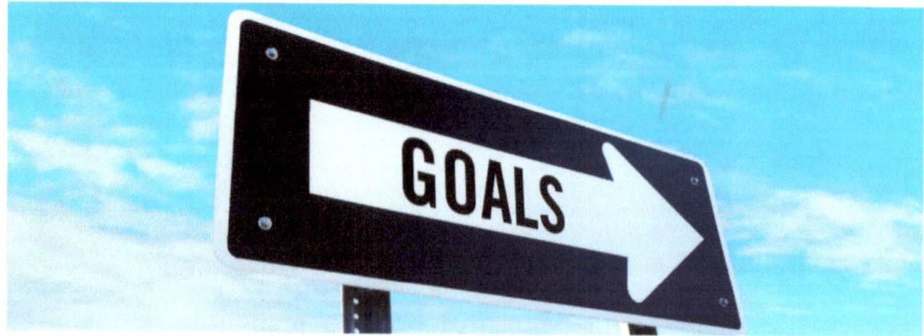

In conclusion, the foundation of a successful health and fitness program lies in the clarity and specificity of your goals. Take the time to define your objectives thoughtfully, and let them serve as the driving force behind your transformative journey towards a healthier, fitter you.

Chapter 2: Your Personalized Health and Fitness Plan

Embarking on a health and fitness program requires more than just enthusiasm; it demands a well-thought-out plan. In this chapter, we'll delve into the essential steps of creating a personalized plan that aligns with your goals, lifestyle, and preferences. A structured plan not only enhances the effectiveness of your efforts but also provides a roadmap for your journey to a healthier and fitter lifestyle.

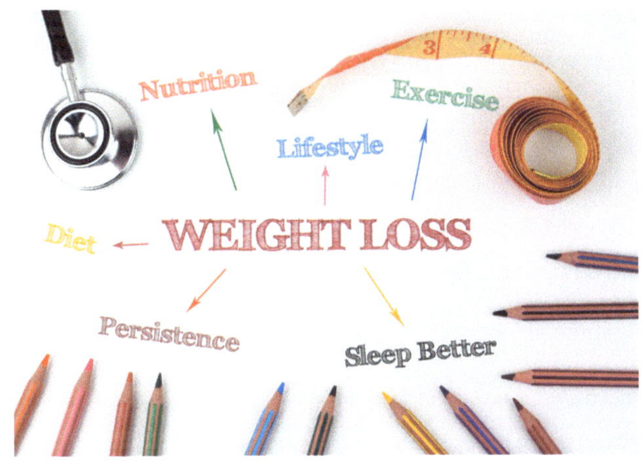

Understanding Your Goals and Preferences

1. **Define Your Objectives**: Before crafting a plan, clearly articulate your health and fitness goals. Whether it's weight loss, muscle gain, increased flexibility, or overall well-being, understanding your objectives is the first step toward a tailored program.

2. **Consider Your Preferences**: Take into account your likes and dislikes when it comes to physical activity and nutrition. Choose exercises and meals that you enjoy, as this increases the likelihood of sticking to your plan in the long run.

Building Your Exercise Routine

1. **Cardiovascular Exercise**: Include cardiovascular activities such as walking, running, cycling, or swimming to improve endurance and heart health. Determine the frequency, duration, and intensity based on your fitness level and goals.

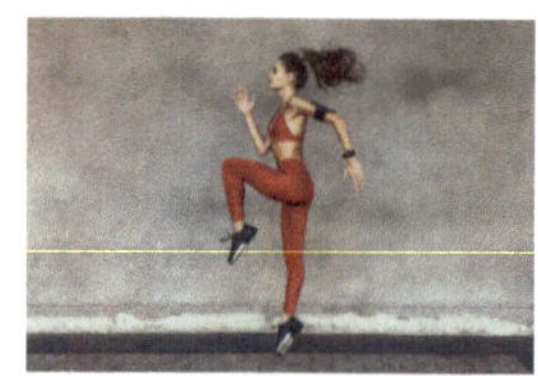

2. **Strength Training**: Integrate strength training exercises to build muscle and boost metabolism. Include a mix of bodyweight exercises, free weights, and resistance training. Aim for a well-rounded approach that targets different muscle groups.

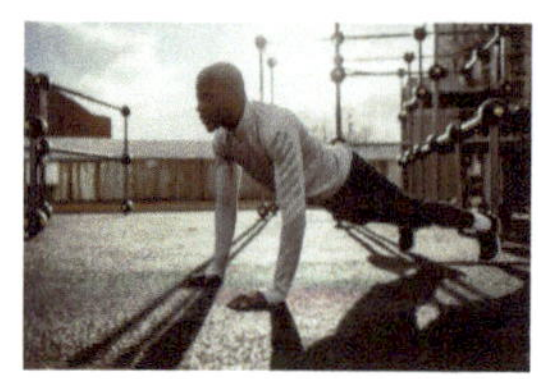

3. **Flexibility and Mobility**: Incorporate stretching, yoga, or Pilates to enhance range of motion, prevent injuries, and promote overall body balance.

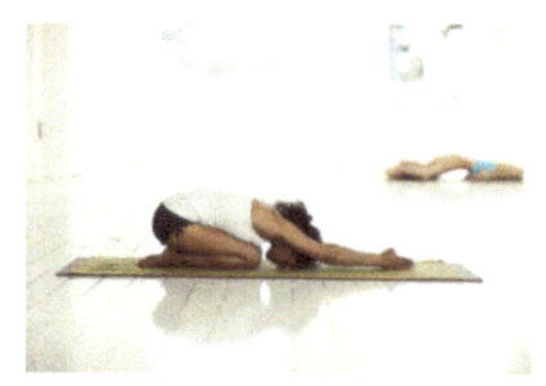

4. **Create a Weekly Schedule**: Plan your workouts in advance and allocate specific time slots for each session. Consistency is key, so choose realistic timeframes that fit into your daily routine.

Nutritional Planning
(more detail in Chapter 4)

1. **Assess Your Dietary Habits**: Take stock of your current eating habits. Identify areas for improvement and recognize any nutritional deficiencies. This self-awareness is crucial for crafting a sustainable and realistic nutrition plan.

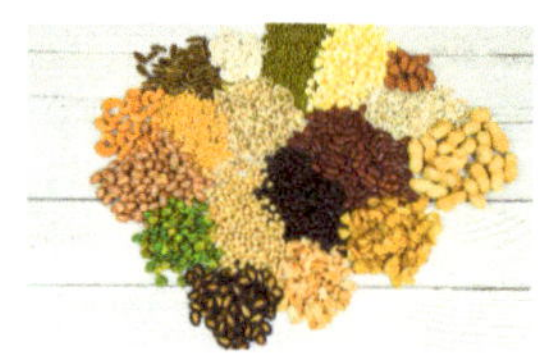

2. **Balanced Nutrition**: Aim for a balanced diet that includes a variety of whole foods. Incorporate lean proteins, colorful fruits and vegetables, whole grains, and healthy fats. Moderation is key, and consider consulting with a nutritionist for personalized advice.

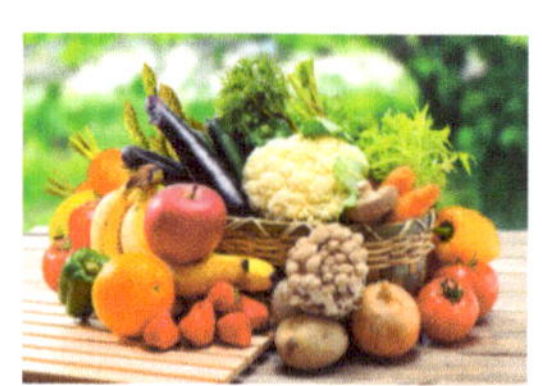

Chapter 3: The Synergy of Cardiovascular & Strength Training

As you embark on your health and fitness journey, it's crucial to recognize the symbiotic relationship between cardiovascular and strength training. Incorporating both elements into your fitness routine not only enhances overall health but also contributes to a well-rounded and effective approach. In this chapter, we'll explore the importance of safely blending cardio and strength training for optimal results.

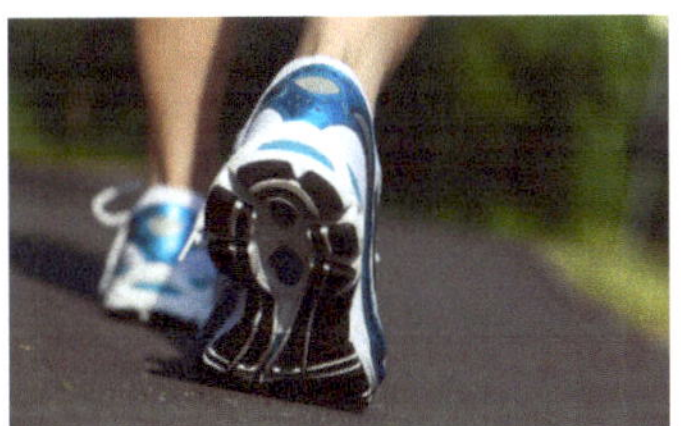 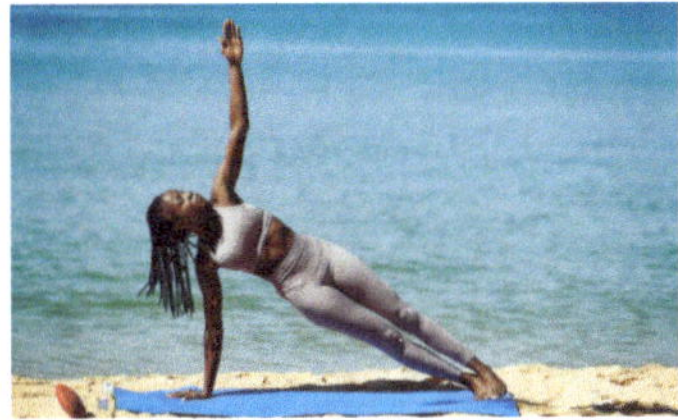

Balancing Heart Health and Muscular Strength

1. **Cardiovascular Benefits**: Cardio exercises, such as walking, running, cycling, and swimming, elevate your heart rate, improving cardiovascular health. They enhance lung capacity, boost circulation, and contribute to better overall endurance.

2. **Strength Training Advantages**: Strength training focuses on building muscle mass and strength. It contributes to increased metabolism, improved bone density, and enhanced functional fitness, reducing the risk of injury and promoting longevity.

Comprehensive Fitness and Weight Management

1. **Effective Caloric Burn**: Cardiovascular workouts are excellent for burning calories and promoting weight loss. Incorporating strength training, you not only burn calories during the session but also continue to burn them post-exercise as your muscles recover and repair.

2. **Muscle Toning and Definition**: Strength training plays a crucial role in sculpting and toning your physique. It helps define muscles, creating a lean and strong appearance. Combining this with cardio prevents excessive muscle loss during weight loss efforts.

Optimizing Workouts for Safety and Efficiency

1. **Proper Warm-Up**: Before engaging in any exercise, it's essential to warm up adequately. A dynamic warm-up prepares your body for the demands of both cardio and strength training, reducing the risk of injuries.

2. **Structured Routine**: Plan your workouts to include a balance of cardio and strength training. This can be achieved through circuit training, interval sessions, or alternating between cardio and strength training days. A well-structured routine ensures that different muscle groups get attention while allowing for sufficient recovery.

3. **Gradual Progression**: Whether you're a beginner or returning to fitness after a break, progress gradually. Avoid pushing yourself too hard, especially in the early stages. Gradual progression minimizes the risk of overtraining and injuries.

Injury Prevention and Joint Health

1. **Joint Support from Strength Training**: Strength training helps build supportive muscles around joints, reducing the risk of injuries. This is especially important for individuals engaging in repetitive movements during cardio exercises.

2. **Correct Form and Technique**: Emphasize proper form and technique in both cardio and strength exercises. This not only maximizes effectiveness but also minimizes the risk of strains, sprains, or joint injuries. Consult with a fitness professional to guide you.

Recovery and Rest Days

1. **Rest for Muscles and Cardiovascular System**: Both cardio and strength training exert stress on your muscles and cardiovascular system. Incorporate rest days into your routine to allow for proper recovery. Adequate rest is essential for muscle repair and overall well-being.

2. **Listen to Your Body**: Pay attention to signs of fatigue or overtraining. If you experience persistent soreness, fatigue, or joint pain, give your body the rest it needs. This prevents burnout and reduces the risk of chronic injuries.

In summary, the synergy of cardio and strength training is a cornerstone of a well-rounded fitness program. By balancing these elements with a focus on safety, gradual progression, and proper recovery, you'll not only enhance your physical health but also set the stage for a sustainable and enjoyable fitness journey.

Chapter 4: Fueling Your Fitness Journey - Crafting an Effective and Safe Nutritional Plan

Embarking on a fitness regimen is not just about exercise; it's a holistic commitment to a healthier lifestyle. A key component of this journey is a well-balanced and safe nutritional plan. In this chapter, we'll explore the importance of nutrition in achieving your fitness goals and provide guidelines for crafting an effective dietary strategy.

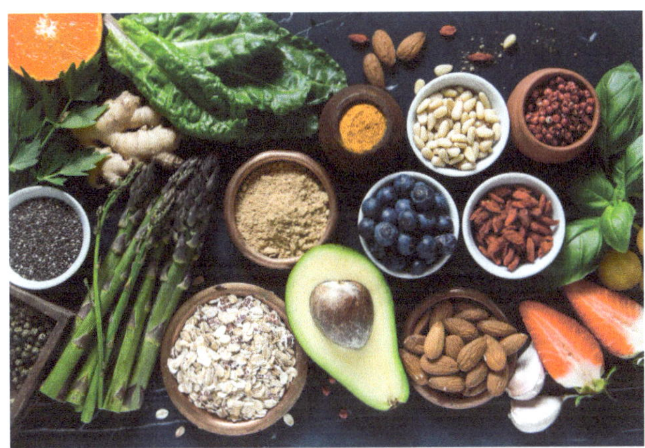

Understanding the Role of Nutrition in Fitness

1. **Fuel for Performance**: Nutrition serves as the fuel that powers your workouts. Consuming the right balance of nutrients ensures optimal energy levels, allowing you to perform at your best during both cardio and strength training sessions.

2. **Muscle Repair and Recovery**: After exercise, your body requires nutrients for muscle repair and recovery. A well-planned nutritional strategy supports these processes, minimizing post-exercise soreness and enhancing overall performance.

Components of an Effective Nutritional Plan

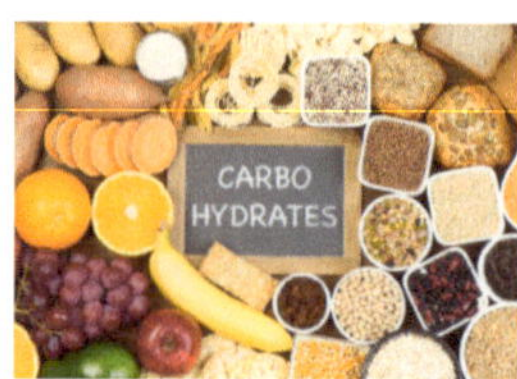

1. **Balanced Macronutrients**: Include a balance of macronutrients in your diet. This includes carbohydrates for energy, proteins for muscle repair, and healthy fats for overall well-being. The proportions may vary based on your specific fitness goals and individual needs.

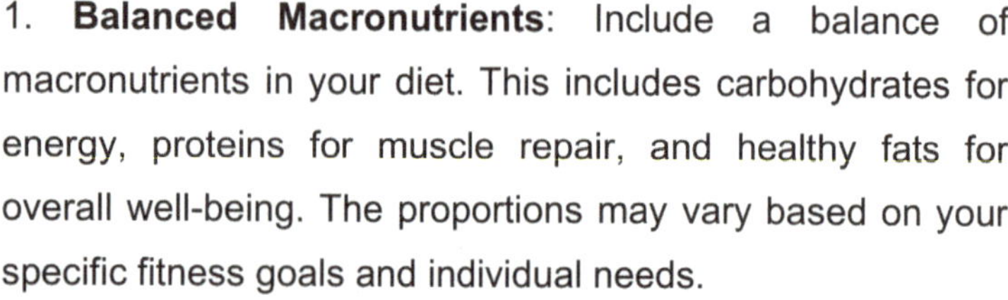

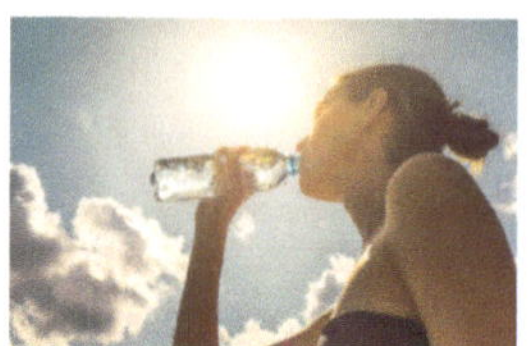

2. **Hydration is Key**: Staying hydrated is crucial for performance and recovery. Water is essential for nutrient transport, temperature regulation, and joint lubrication. Ensure you drink an adequate amount of water throughout the day, especially before, during, and after workouts.

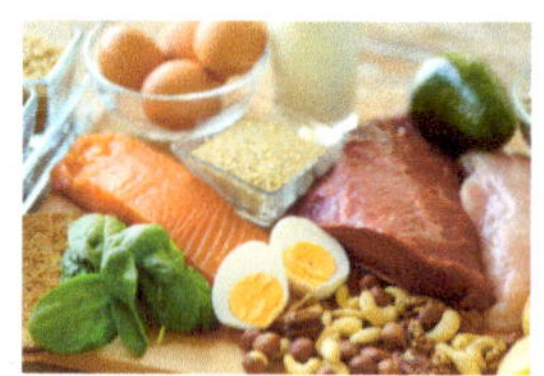

3. **Whole Foods and Nutrient Density**: Prioritize whole, nutrient-dense foods. These include fruits, vegetables, lean proteins, whole grains, and healthy fats. These foods not only provide essential nutrients but also support overall health and weight management.

Meal Timing and Pre-Workout Nutrition

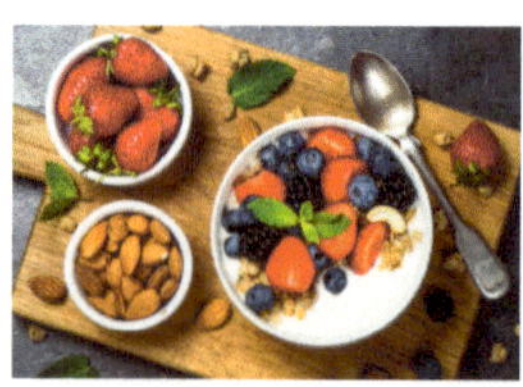

1. **Pre-Workout Fuel**: Consume a balanced meal or snack one to two hours before your workout. This should include carbohydrates for energy and a moderate amount of protein. Examples include a banana with nut butter, Greek yogurt with berries, or a small chicken and vegetable wrap.

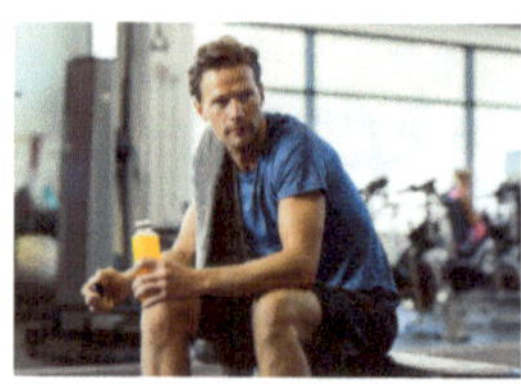

2. **Post-Workout Nutrition**: Refuel your body with a combination of protein and carbohydrates within 30 minutes of finishing your workout. This aids in muscle recovery and replenishes glycogen stores. Options include a protein shake, chocolate milk, or a balanced meal with lean protein and whole grains.

Portion Control and Mindful Eating 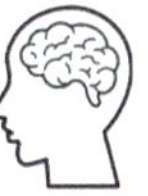

1. **Listen to Your Body**: Pay attention to hunger and fullness cues. Eating mindfully helps prevent overeating and promotes a healthier relationship with food. Chew your food slowly, savoring each bite, and be conscious of portion sizes.

2. **Regular, Balanced Meals**: Aim for regular, balanced meals throughout the day. This helps maintain stable energy levels and prevents excessive hunger, reducing the likelihood of unhealthy snacking.

Individualization and Professional Guidance

1. **Tailor Your Plan**: Recognize that nutritional needs vary among individuals. Consider your age, gender, activity level, and specific fitness goals when crafting your plan. What works for one person may not be suitable for another.

2. **Consult with Nutrition Experts**: If you're unsure about creating a personalized nutritional plan, consult with registered dietitians or nutritionists. They can provide expert guidance based on your individual needs, ensuring that your plan is safe, effective, and aligned with your fitness goals.

Consistency and Long-Term Sustainability

1. **Build Habits Gradually**: Implement changes gradually to allow for better adaptation. Building sustainable habits over time increases the likelihood of long-term success in both your fitness and nutritional endeavors.

2. **Celebrate Progress**: Acknowledge and celebrate your nutritional achievements along the way. This positive reinforcement contributes to the overall enjoyment of your fitness journey.

In conclusion, an effective and safe nutritional plan is a cornerstone of a successful fitness regimen. By understanding the role of nutrition, focusing on balanced macronutrients, and tailoring your approach to individual needs, you'll fuel your body for optimal performance and set the stage for a healthier lifestyle throughout the new year and beyond.

Chapter 5: The Power of Consistency and Rest in Your Fitness Journey

Embarking on a fitness regimen is an admirable commitment to your well-being. However, the journey to a healthier lifestyle is not just about intense workouts; it's about embracing consistency and recognizing the essential role of rest in achieving sustainable results. In this chapter, we'll explore the impact of consistency and rest on your fitness journey.

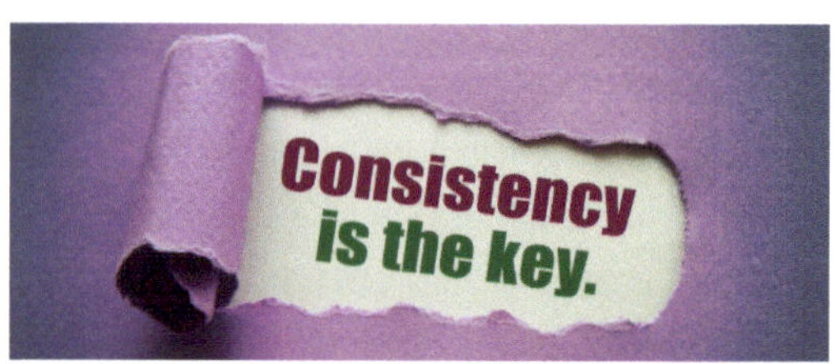

Consistency: The Key to Long-Term Success

1. **Establishing Habits**: Consistency is the foundation upon which healthy habits are built. Regular exercise and adherence to a nutritional plan become ingrained in your routine, making them more sustainable over time.

2. **Incremental Progress**: Fitness is a journey, not a destination. Consistent effort, even in small increments, leads to cumulative progress. Whether it's gradual strength improvements, increased endurance, or better flexibility, each workout contributes to your overall well-being.

3. **Mental and Emotional Benefits:** Consistency extends beyond physical changes. Regular exercise has proven mental and emotional benefits, including stress reduction, improved mood, and enhanced cognitive function. Positive effects compound with consistent effort.

4. **Building Self-Discipline**: Consistency cultivates self-discipline. Committing to your fitness regimen, even on days when motivation is low, strengthens your self-discipline and resilience, fostering a mindset of dedication and determination.

The Importance of Rest and Recovery

1. **Muscle Repair and Growth**: Rest days are not a sign of weakness; they are an integral part of the fitness journey. During rest, your muscles repair and grow stronger. Continuous, high-intensity workouts without adequate rest can lead to overtraining, fatigue, and increased risk of injury.

2. **Preventing Burnout**: Burnout is a real concern in the fitness world. Consistent, intense training without sufficient rest can lead to physical and mental exhaustion. Incorporating rest days helps prevent burnout, ensuring that your enthusiasm and energy levels remain high.

3. **Balancing Hormones**: Intense workouts elevate stress hormones like cortisol. Adequate rest and recovery help balance these hormones, promoting overall hormonal health. This balance is crucial for optimal fitness progress and general well-being.

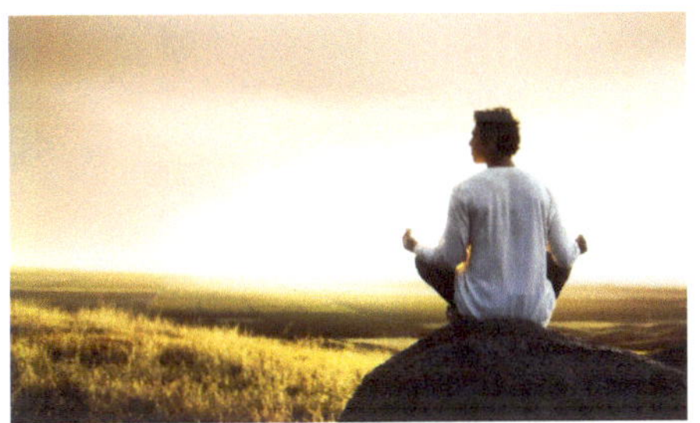 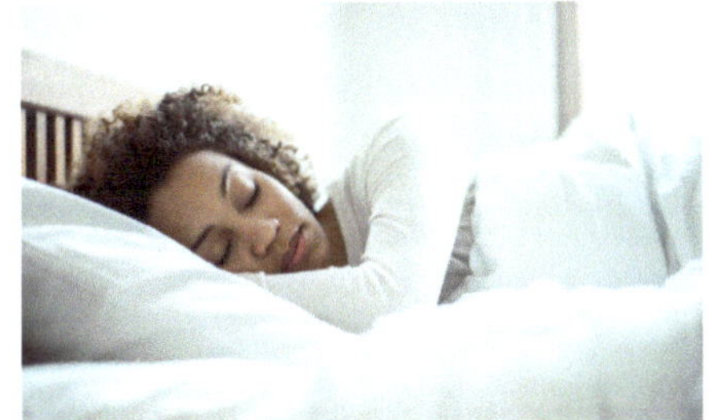

Quality Sleep as Part of Rest

1. **Recharge with Sleep**: Sleep is a vital component of rest and recovery. Aim for 7-9 hours of quality sleep each night. During sleep, the body undergoes essential processes that support physical and mental health, including muscle repair, hormone regulation, and cognitive consolidation.

2. **Sleep and Performance**: Insufficient sleep negatively impacts performance, cognitive function, and the body's ability to recover. Prioritize sleep as an integral part of your fitness routine, recognizing its direct influence on your overall well-being.

Strategies for Consistency and Rest

1. **Schedule Rest Days**: Plan regular rest days into your weekly routine. This deliberate scheduling ensures that rest is a proactive part of your fitness plan rather than a reaction to fatigue or injury.

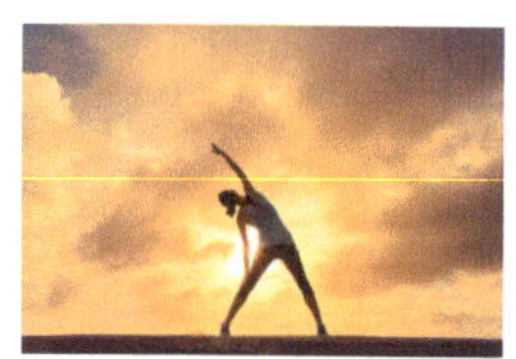

2. **Active Recovery**: On rest days, consider engaging in light activities such as walking, yoga, or stretching. Active recovery promotes blood circulation, reduces muscle stiffness, and aids in overall recovery without the intensity of regular workouts.

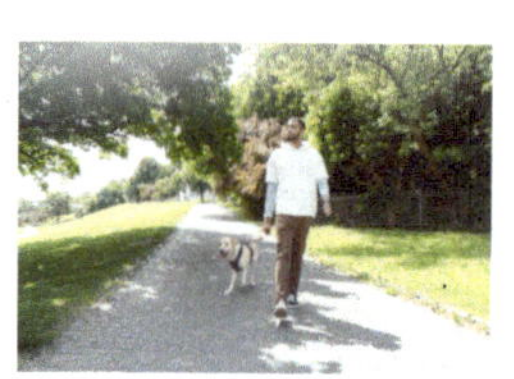

3. **Listen to Your Body**: Pay attention to your body's signals. If you're feeling fatigued, sore, or unusually low in energy, it may be a sign that your body needs additional rest. Listen to these cues and adjust your workout intensity.

Professional Guidance and Support

1. **Consultation with Experts**: If you're unsure about the balance between consistency and rest in your fitness plan, seek guidance from fitness professionals. Personal trainers or fitness coaches can provide personalized advice, helping you tailor your routine.

2. **Incorporate Variety**: Consistency doesn't mean monotony. Incorporate variety into your workouts to keep things interesting. This can involve trying different exercises, classes, or outdoor activities. Variety not only prevents boredom but also engages different muscle groups.

In conclusion, the success of your fitness journey lies in the delicate balance between consistency and rest. Embrace the power of regular, dedicated effort while recognizing the importance of allowing your body to recover. By incorporating these principles into your fitness regimen, you'll pave the way for sustainable progress, improved well-being, and a positive relationship with your health throughout the new year and beyond.

Chapter 6: Motivation and Positivity in Your Fitness Odyssey

Embarking on a fitness regimen signifies a commitment to self-improvement and well-being. While the initial excitement is powerful, sustaining motivation and maintaining a positive mindset are integral to long-term success. In this chapter, we'll explore the importance of staying motivated and positive throughout your fitness journey.

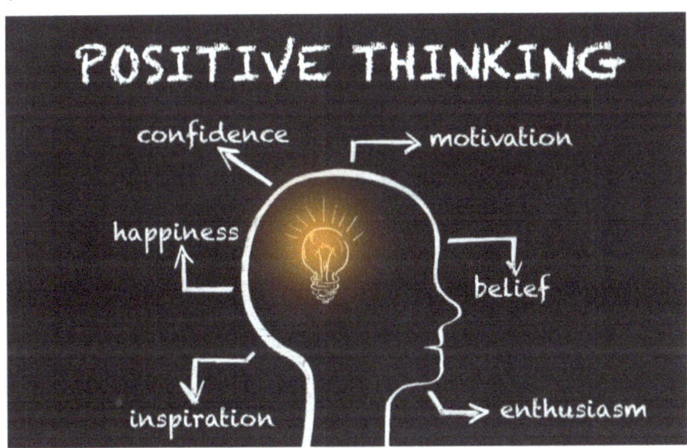

Cultivating a Positive Mindset

1. **Embracing Challenges**: A positive mindset is your armor against challenges. Instead of viewing obstacles as insurmountable, see them as opportunities for growth. Challenges are an inherent part of any fitness journey, and a positive outlook helps you navigate with resilience.

2. **Celebrating Small Wins**: Acknowledge and celebrate every achievement, no matter how small. Whether it's completing an extra set of exercises, running an extra mile, or making healthier food choices, recognizing victories reinforces your commitment and boosts morale.

3. **Focusing on Progress, Not Perfection**: Strive for progress, not perfection. Understand that fitness is a continuous journey of improvement, and it's okay to have setbacks. A positive mindset allows you to learn from challenges and keep moving forward.

The Role of Motivation in Fitness

1. **Initiating Action**: Motivation is the driving force that propels you into action. It's the spark that ignites your desire to make positive changes in your life. Recognize and harness this initial motivation to kickstart your fitness journey.

2. **Sustaining Momentum**: While the initial burst of motivation is potent, it's essential to cultivate strategies for sustaining momentum. Long-term success in fitness relies on consistent effort, and motivation serves as the fuel that keeps you going, even on challenging days.

Strategies for Staying Motivated

1. **Set Realistic and Achievable Goals**: Goals provide direction and motivation. Ensure they are realistic, specific, and achievable within a given timeframe. Break down larger goals into smaller, manageable milestones, making it easier to track progress and stay motivated.

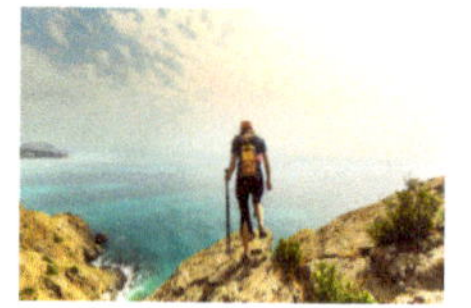

2. **Find Enjoyable Activities**: Engage in activities you enjoy. Whether it's a favorite sport, dance class, or outdoors, incorporating enjoyable elements into your fitness routine makes the journey more sustainable and fulfilling.

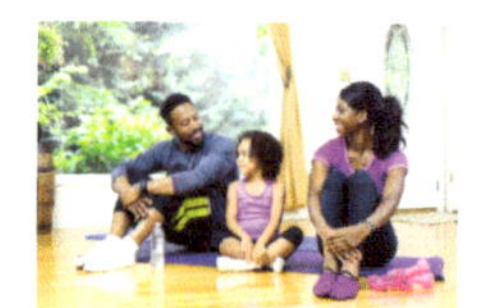

3. **Variety in Workouts**: Keep your workouts varied to prevent monotony. Trying new exercises, classes, or outdoor activities not only challenges your body in different ways but also keeps your interest alive.

4. **Create a Support System**: Share your fitness goals with friends, family, or a workout buddy. Having a support system provides encouragement and accountability. Celebrate successes together and lean on each other during challenging times.

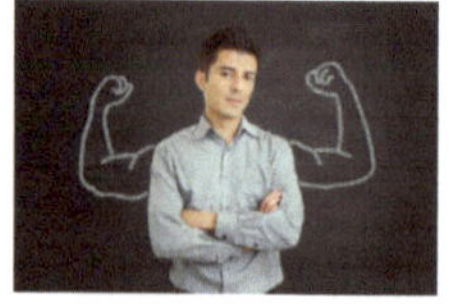

Overcoming Challenges with Positivity

1. **Mindful Self-Talk**: Pay attention to your internal dialogue. Replace negative self-talk with positive affirmations. Instead of focusing on limitations, emphasize your strengths and the progress you've made.

2. **Learn from Setbacks**: View setbacks as opportunities to learn and grow. Instead of dwelling on a missed workout or an indulgent meal, reflect on what led to the setback and use it as a stepping stone for improvement.

Mind-Body Connection

1. **Mindfulness Practices**: Incorporate mindfulness practices such as meditation or yoga into your routine. These practices not only contribute to mental well-being but also enhance the mind-body connection, fostering a holistic approach to fitness.

2. **Visualize Success**: Picture yourself achieving your fitness goals. Visualization can be a powerful motivator, helping you stay focused on the positive outcomes of your efforts.

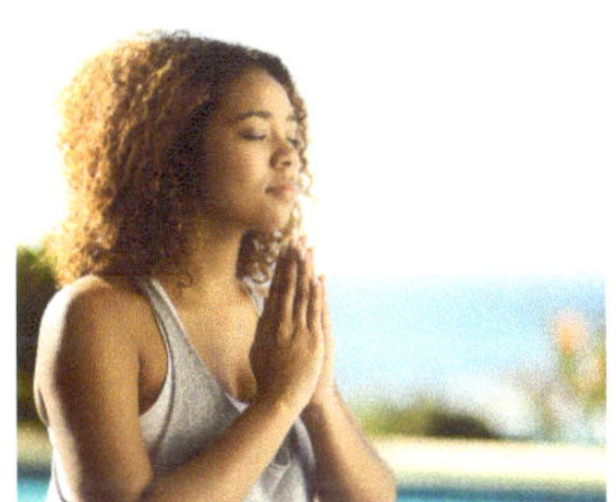 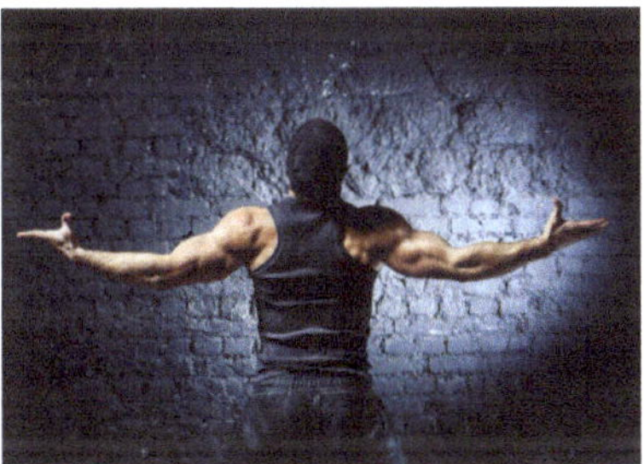

Seeking Inspiration

1. **Follow Fitness Role Models**: Follow fitness influencers, athletes, or role models who inspire you. Their journeys and achievements can serve as a source of motivation and provide valuable insights into overcoming challenges.

2. **Educate Yourself**: Learn about the benefits of exercise, nutrition, and overall well-being. Understanding the positive impact of your efforts on your health can be a powerful motivator.

In conclusion, the importance of staying motivated and positive in your fitness journey cannot be overstated. By understanding the role of motivation, cultivating a positive mindset, and implementing strategies to stay inspired, you'll pave the way for a fulfilling and successful fitness regimen throughout the new year and beyond.

Chapter 7: Embracing a Healthier You - Closing Thoughts on Your Fitness Journey

Congratulations on embarking on the transformative journey of starting a health and fitness program. This endeavor reflects your commitment to self-improvement, well-being, and a healthier lifestyle. As you conclude this comprehensive guide, let's reflect on the key principles that will guide you towards lasting success in your fitness journey.

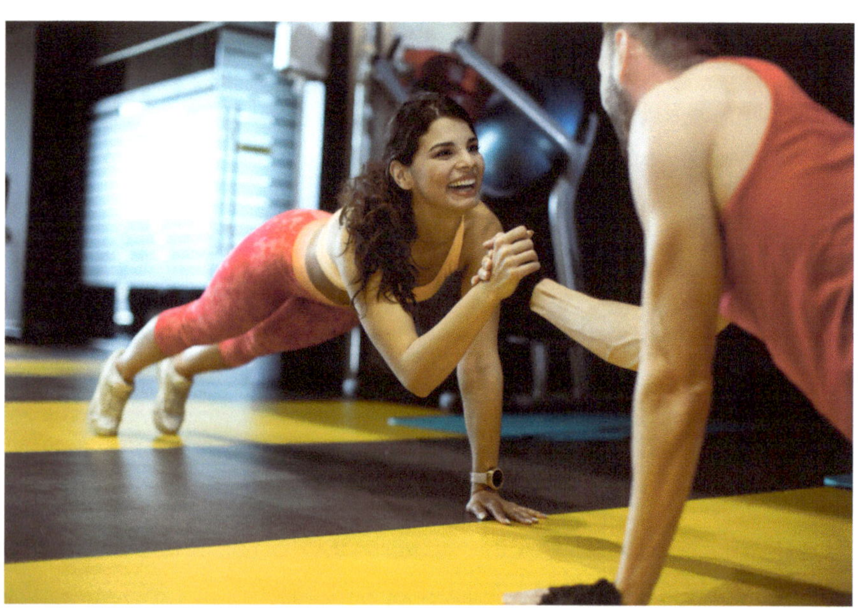

Goal Setting and Planning

Clear and realistic goal-setting is your roadmap to success. Whether it's weight loss, muscle gain, or improved endurance, well-defined goals provide direction. Yet, it's equally important to embrace adaptability. Life is dynamic, and your fitness plan should evolve with your changing circumstances.

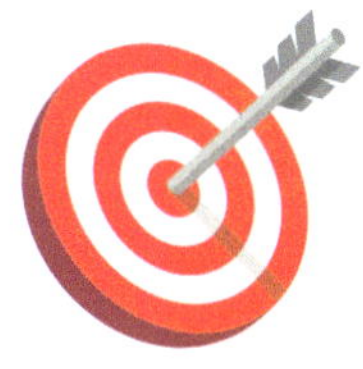

Balancing Cardio and Strength Training

The synergy between cardiovascular and strength training is a potent combination for comprehensive fitness. By safely blending these elements into your routine, you're not only improving your cardiovascular health but also building strength, muscle tone, and resilience.

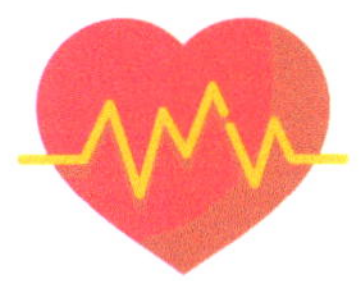

Nutrition as Fuel for Success

Your body is a reflection of what you feed it. A well-crafted nutritional plan is the fuel that powers your fitness journey. Prioritize balanced macronutrients, stay hydrated, and embrace the concept of nourishing your body for optimal performance.

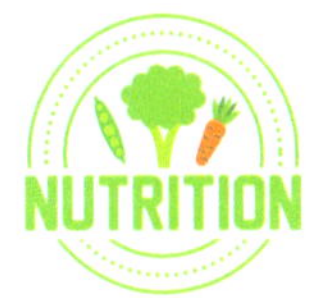

Consistency, Rest, and Recovery

Consistency is the bedrock of success, but it should be complemented by rest and recovery. Overtraining can impede progress and lead to burnout. Embrace the power of rest days, quality sleep, and listen to your body's signals for a sustainable and effective fitness regimen.

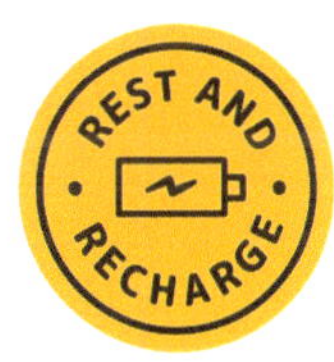

Staying Motivated and Positive

Motivation and positivity are the driving forces that will carry you through the inevitable challenges of your fitness journey. Cultivate a positive mindset, celebrate small wins, and use setbacks as stepping stones for growth. Stay connected with your motivation, and let it fuel your ongoing commitment to a healthier lifestyle.

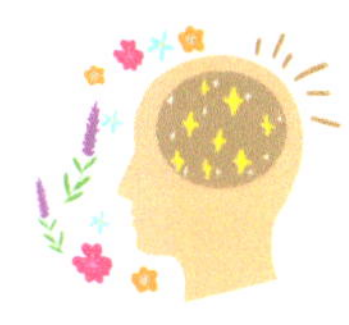

Building Lasting Habits for a Healthier Future

Remember that your fitness journey is a marathon, not a sprint. Aim to build lasting habits that seamlessly integrate into your lifestyle. By consistently prioritizing your health, you're creating a foundation for a future filled with vitality, energy, and overall well-being. As you close this chapter and step into your fitness journey, carry with you the knowledge, motivation, and commitment you've cultivated. Embrace the challenges as opportunities for growth, celebrate your victories, and stay resilient in the face of setbacks. Your health is a lifelong investment, and with each step, you're moving closer to becoming the best version of yourself. Here's to a healthier, fitter, and more vibrant you. Cheers to your well-being and the exciting journey that lies ahead!

WEEK 1 GOAL SETTING

SPECIFIC TARGETS

WORKOUT DAYS/TIME

MEAL PLANNING

CARDIO EXERCISE & DAY

STRENGTH EXERCISE & DAY

FLEXIBILITY EXERCISE & DAY

SMALL VICTORIES

REST DAY PLAN

HEALTHY FOODS

KEEP GOING!

WEEK 2 GOAL SETTING

SPECIFIC TARGETS

WORKOUT DAYS/TIME

MEAL PLANNING

CARDIO EXERCISE & DAY

STRENGTH EXERCISE & DAY

FLEXIBILITY EXERCISE & DAY

SMALL VICTORIES

- ◯
- ◯
- ◯
- ◯
- ◯
- ◯
- ◯

REST DAY PLAN

♥

HEALTHY FOODS

KEEP GOING!

WEEK 3 GOAL SETTING

SPECIFIC TARGETS

WORKOUT DAYS/TIME

MEAL PLANNING

CARDIO EXERCISE & DAY

STRENGTH EXERCISE & DAY

FLEXIBILITY EXERCISE & DAY

SMALL VICTORIES

REST DAY PLAN

HEALTHY FOODS

KEEP GOING!

WEEK 4 GOAL SETTING

SPECIFIC TARGETS

WORKOUT DAYS/TIME

MEAL PLANNING

CARDIO EXERCISE & DAY

STRENGTH EXERCISE & DAY

FLEXIBILITY EXERCISE & DAY

SMALL VICTORIES

- ◯
- ◯
- ◯
- ◯
- ◯
- ◯
- ◯

REST DAY PLAN

HEALTHY FOODS

KEEP GOING!

WEEK 5 GOAL SETTING

SPECIFIC TARGETS

WORKOUT DAYS/TIME

MEAL PLANNING

CARDIO EXERCISE & DAY

STRENGTH EXERCISE & DAY

FLEXIBILITY EXERCISE & DAY

SMALL VICTORIES

- ◯
- ◯
- ◯
- ◯
- ◯
- ◯
- ◯

REST DAY PLAN

♥

HEALTHY FOODS

KEEP GOING!

WEEK 6 GOAL SETTING

SPECIFIC TARGETS

WORKOUT DAYS/TIME

MEAL PLANNING

CARDIO EXERCISE & DAY

STRENGTH EXERCISE & DAY

FLEXIBILITY EXERCISE & DAY

SMALL VICTORIES

- ◯
- ◯
- ◯
- ◯
- ◯
- ◯
- ◯

REST DAY PLAN

HEALTHY FOODS

KEEP GOING!

WEEK 7
GOAL SETTING

SPECIFIC TARGETS

WORKOUT DAYS/TIME

MEAL PLANNING

CARDIO EXERCISE & DAY

STRENGTH EXERCISE & DAY

FLEXIBILITY EXERCISE & DAY

SMALL VICTORIES

- ○
- ○
- ○
- ○
- ○
- ○
- ○

REST DAY PLAN

♥

HEALTHY FOODS

KEEP GOING!

WEEK 8
GOAL SETTING

SPECIFIC TARGETS

WORKOUT DAYS/TIME

MEAL PLANNING

CARDIO EXERCISE & DAY

STRENGTH EXERCISE & DAY

FLEXIBILITY EXERCISE & DAY

SMALL VICTORIES

REST DAY PLAN

HEALTHY FOODS

KEEP GOING!

SPECIFIC TARGETS

WORKOUT DAYS/TIME

MEAL PLANNING

CARDIO EXERCISE & DAY

STRENGTH EXERCISE & DAY

FLEXIBILITY EXERCISE & DAY

SMALL VICTORIES

- ◯
- ◯
- ◯
- ◯
- ◯
- ◯
- ◯

REST DAY PLAN

♥

HEALTHY FOODS

KEEP GOING!

WEEK 10
GOAL SETTING

SPECIFIC TARGETS

WORKOUT DAYS/TIME

MEAL PLANNING

CARDIO EXERCISE
& DAY

STRENGTH EXERCISE
& DAY

FLEXIBILITY
EXERCISE & DAY

SMALL VICTORIES

REST DAY PLAN

HEALTHY FOODS

KEEP GOING!